Introducing an exciting new teaching tool

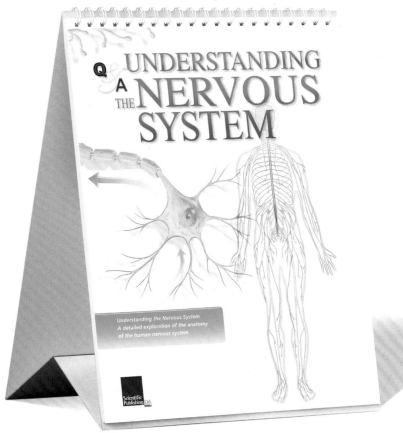

Understanding the Nervous System flip chart

This beautifully illustrated flip chart study guide is an ideal reference tool for home, library, or patient education. Each flip chart provides an in-depth, yet easily accessible exploration of the featured topic, complete with clear, concise text and original artwork of anatomy, physiological processes and disease pathology.

- **Portable, fully illustrated flip chart design**
- **Easy-to-read Question & Answer format**
- **Ideal for home, library and office**

Pages from Understanding the Nervous System flip chart

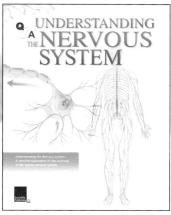
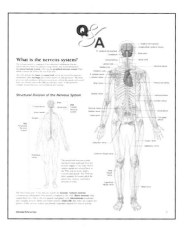
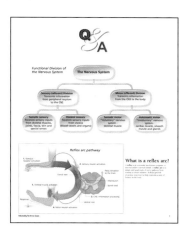

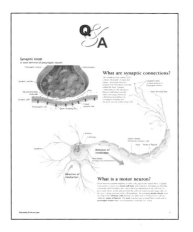
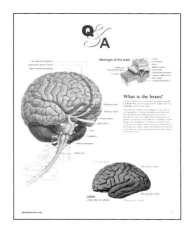
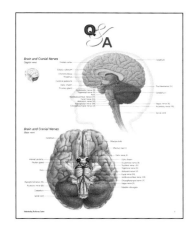
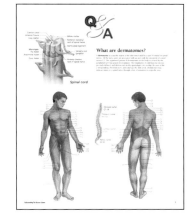
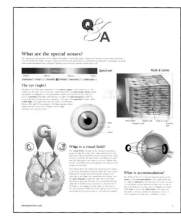

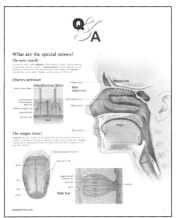
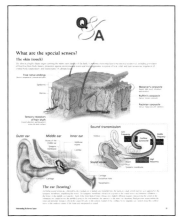
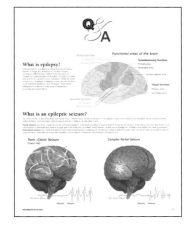
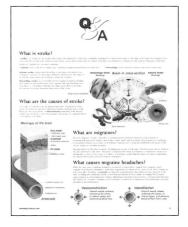
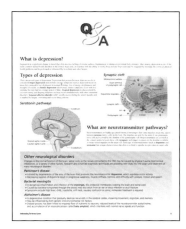

Other titles in our anatomical flip chart series

Understanding Arthritis Item# 1052F	ISBN-13: 978-1-932922-28-8	ISBN-10: 1-932922-28-8
Understanding Cholesterol Item# 1651F	ISBN-13: 978-1-932922-33-2	ISBN-10: 1-932922-33-4
Understanding Hypertension Item# 1450F	ISBN-13: 978-1-932922-30-1	ISBN-10: 1-932922-30-X
Understanding the Digestive System Item# 1500F	ISBN-13: 978-1-932922-31-8	ISBN-10: 1-932922-31-8
Understanding Hepatitis Item# 1950F	ISBN-13: 978-1-932922-34-9	ISBN-10: 1-932922-34-2
Understanding Skin Item# 2500F	ISBN-13: 978-1-932922-35-6	ISBN-10: 1-932922-35-0
Understanding COPD Item# 1351F	ISBN-13: 978-1-932922-29-5	ISBN-10: 1-932922-29-6
Understanding Diabetes Item# 1650F	ISBN-13: 978-1-932922-32-5	ISBN-10: 1-932922-32-6

ISBN-13: 978-1-932922-87-5
ISBN-10: 1-932922-87-3

51595

Understanding the Nervous System Item# 2700F   ISBN-13: 978-1-932922-87-5   ©2010 Scientific Publishing Ltd. Elk Grove Village, IL USA www.scientificpublishing.com   Printed in USA

9 781932 922875

Q & A

UNDERSTANDING THE NERVOUS SYSTEM

Understanding the Nervous System — A detailed look at the anatomy of the human nervous system, including its common diseases and disorders.

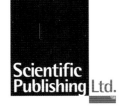

Scientific Publishing Ltd.

First Edition: March 2010

Published in the United States by
Scientific Publishing Ltd.
129 Joey Drive
Elk Grove Village, IL 60007

Individual chart titles are available at www.scientificpublishing.com

Understanding The Nervous System
Item# 2700F
ISBN-13: 978-1-932922-87-5
ISBN-10: 1-932922-87-3

Printed and bound in USA

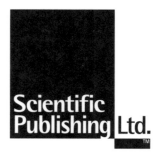

Q&A

What is the nervous system?

The nervous system is composed of two integrated subdivisions that are responsible for conducting and processing sensory and motor information: the **central nervous system** (CNS) and the **peripheral nervous system** (PNS), which connects the CNS to the rest of the body.

The CNS includes the **brain** and **spinal cord**, which are covered by protective membranes called **meninges** (dura mater, arachnoid and pia mater). The brain processes and coordinates all neural signals received from the spinal cord as well as its own nerves, such as the olfactory and optic nerves. It also performs complex mental functions such as thinking and learning.

Structural division of the nervous system

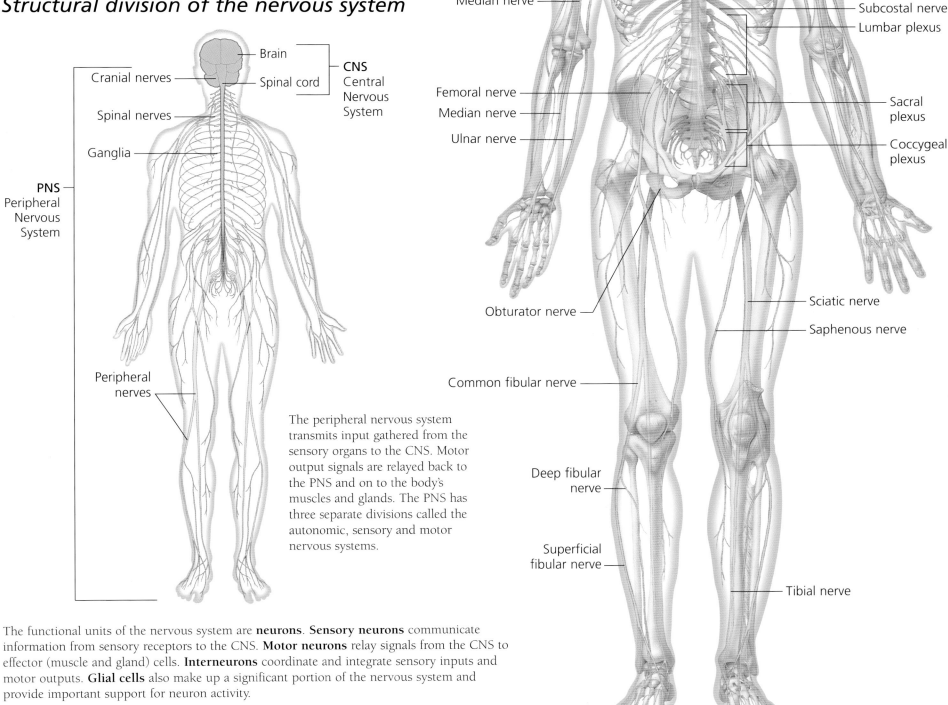

Brain
Cranial nerves
Spinal cord
CNS Central Nervous System
Spinal nerves
Ganglia
PNS Peripheral Nervous System
Peripheral nerves

The peripheral nervous system transmits input gathered from the sensory organs to the CNS. Motor output signals are relayed back to the PNS and on to the body's muscles and glands. The PNS has three separate divisions called the autonomic, sensory and motor nervous systems.

R. cerebral hemisphere
L. cerebral hemisphere
Longitudinal cerebral fissure
Cerebellum
Brain stem
Cervical plexus
Spinal cord
Lateral cord
Brachial plexus
Medial cord
Posterior cord
R. phrenic nerve
L. phrenic nerve
Intercostal nerves
Median nerve
Subcostal nerve
Lumbar plexus
Femoral nerve
Median nerve
Ulnar nerve
Sacral plexus
Coccygeal plexus
Obturator nerve
Sciatic nerve
Saphenous nerve
Common fibular nerve
Deep fibular nerve
Superficial fibular nerve
Tibial nerve

The functional units of the nervous system are **neurons**. **Sensory neurons** communicate information from sensory receptors to the CNS. **Motor neurons** relay signals from the CNS to effector (muscle and gland) cells. **Interneurons** coordinate and integrate sensory inputs and motor outputs. **Glial cells** also make up a significant portion of the nervous system and provide important support for neuron activity.

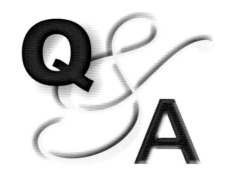

Functional division of the nervous system

The Nervous System

Sensory (afferent) division
Transmits information from peripheral receptors to the CNS

Motor (efferent) division
Transmits information from the CNS to the body

Somatic sensory
Receives sensory inputs from skeletal muscles, joints, fascia, skin and special senses

Visceral sensory
Receives sensory inputs from blood vessels and organs

Somatic motor
"Voluntary" nervous system — skeletal muscle

Autonomic motor
"Involuntary" nervous system — cardiac muscle, smooth muscle and glands

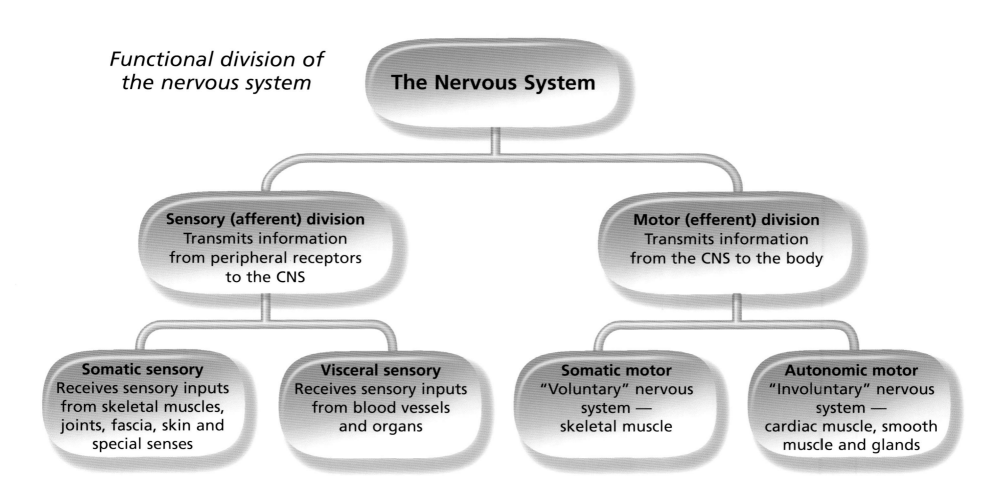

Reflex arc pathway

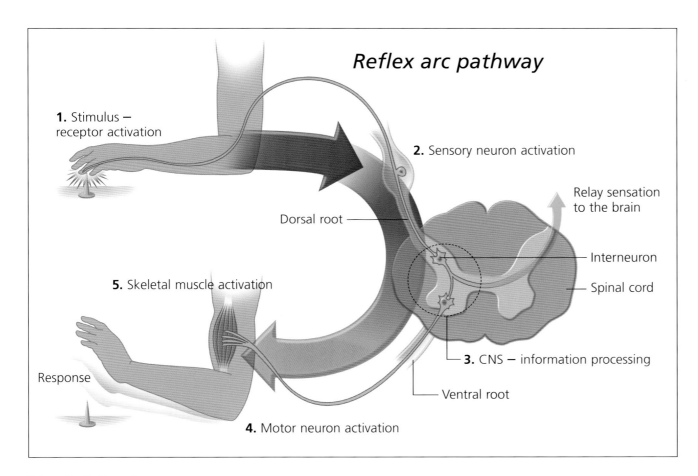

1. Stimulus — receptor activation

2. Sensory neuron activation

Relay sensation to the brain

Dorsal root

Interneuron

Spinal cord

5. Skeletal muscle activation

3. CNS — information processing

Response

Ventral root

4. Motor neuron activation

What is a reflex arc?

A **reflex** is an automatic involuntary response to internal and/or external stimuli. A **reflex arc** is a simple and quick type of nerve pathway from sensory to motor neurons. Reflexes provide protective responses to help maintain a state of balance in the body.

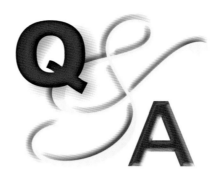

Synaptic knob
or axon terminal of presynaptic neuron

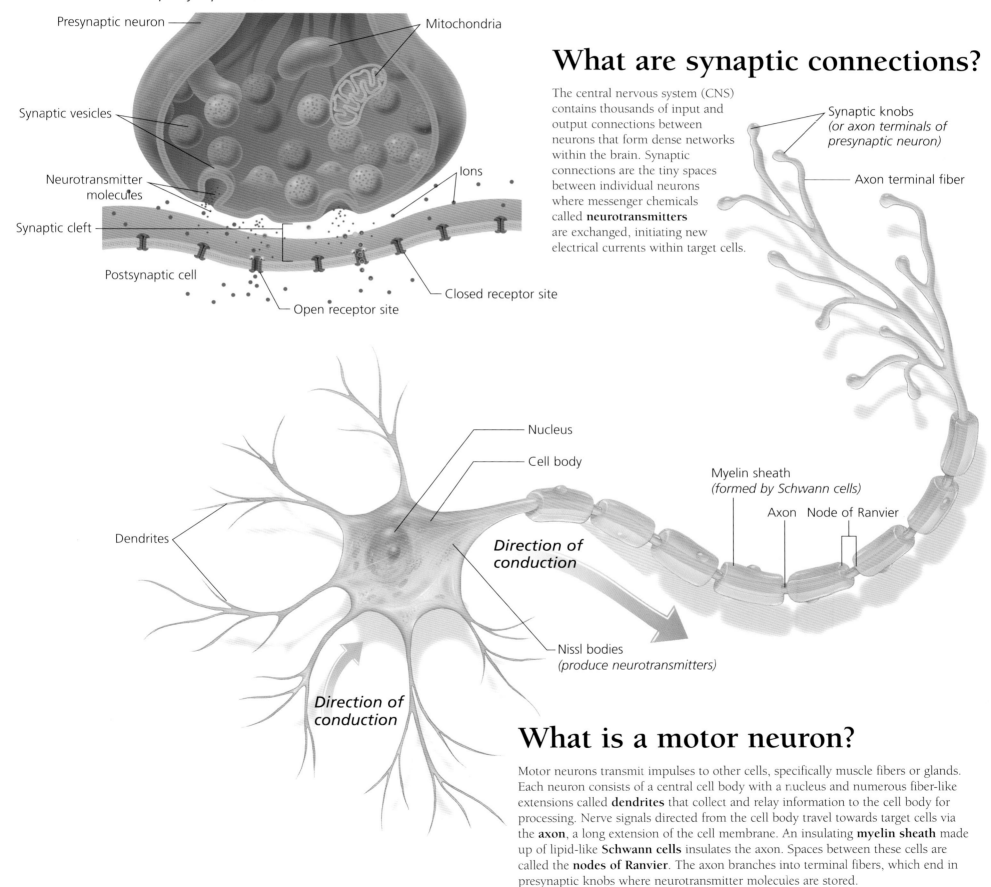

Presynaptic neuron

Mitochondria

Synaptic vesicles

Neurotransmitter molecules

Ions

Synaptic cleft

Postsynaptic cell

Open receptor site

Closed receptor site

What are synaptic connections?

The central nervous system (CNS) contains thousands of input and output connections between neurons that form dense networks within the brain. Synaptic connections are the tiny spaces between individual neurons where messenger chemicals called **neurotransmitters** are exchanged, initiating new electrical currents within target cells.

Synaptic knobs
(or axon terminals of presynaptic neuron)

Axon terminal fiber

Nucleus

Cell body

Myelin sheath
(formed by Schwann cells)

Axon   Node of Ranvier

Dendrites

Direction of conduction

Nissl bodies
(produce neurotransmitters)

Direction of conduction

What is a motor neuron?

Motor neurons transmit impulses to other cells, specifically muscle fibers or glands. Each neuron consists of a central cell body with a nucleus and numerous fiber-like extensions called **dendrites** that collect and relay information to the cell body for processing. Nerve signals directed from the cell body travel towards target cells via the **axon**, a long extension of the cell membrane. An insulating **myelin sheath** made up of lipid-like **Schwann cells** insulates the axon. Spaces between these cells are called the **nodes of Ranvier**. The axon branches into terminal fibers, which end in presynaptic knobs where neurotransmitter molecules are stored.

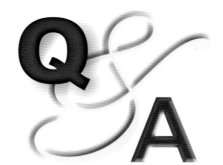

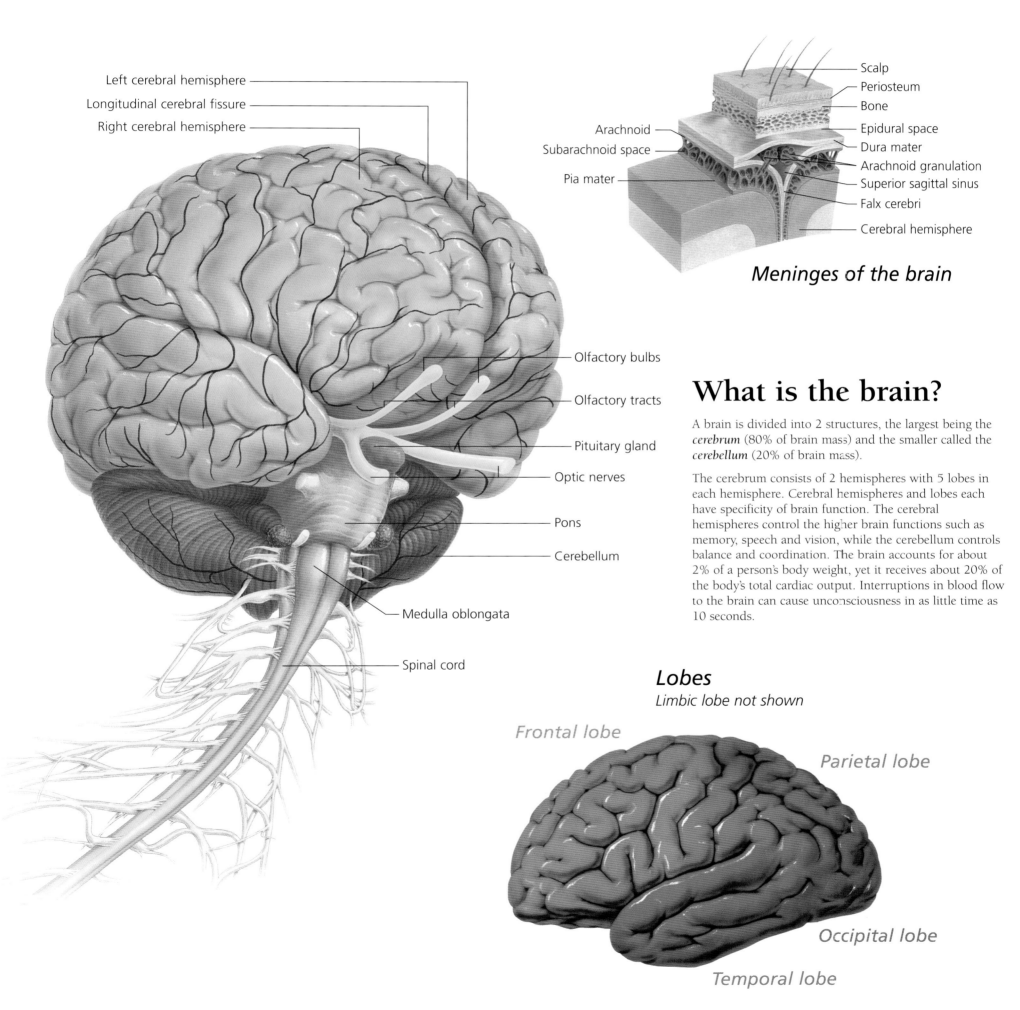

Left cerebral hemisphere

Longitudinal cerebral fissure

Right cerebral hemisphere

Olfactory bulbs

Olfactory tracts

Pituitary gland

Optic nerves

Pons

Cerebellum

Medulla oblongata

Spinal cord

Scalp

Periosteum

Bone

Arachnoid

Epidural space

Subarachnoid space

Dura mater

Arachnoid granulation

Pia mater

Superior sagittal sinus

Falx cerebri

Cerebral hemisphere

Meninges of the brain

What is the brain?

A brain is divided into 2 structures, the largest being the *cerebrum* (80% of brain mass) and the smaller called the *cerebellum* (20% of brain mass).

The cerebrum consists of 2 hemispheres with 5 lobes in each hemisphere. Cerebral hemispheres and lobes each have specificity of brain function. The cerebral hemispheres control the higher brain functions such as memory, speech and vision, while the cerebellum controls balance and coordination. The brain accounts for about 2% of a person's body weight, yet it receives about 20% of the body's total cardiac output. Interruptions in blood flow to the brain can cause unconsciousness in as little time as 10 seconds.

Lobes
Limbic lobe not shown

Frontal lobe

Parietal lobe

Occipital lobe

Temporal lobe

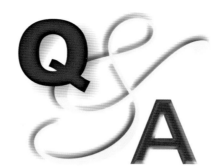

Q & A

Brain and cranial nerves
(Sagittal view)

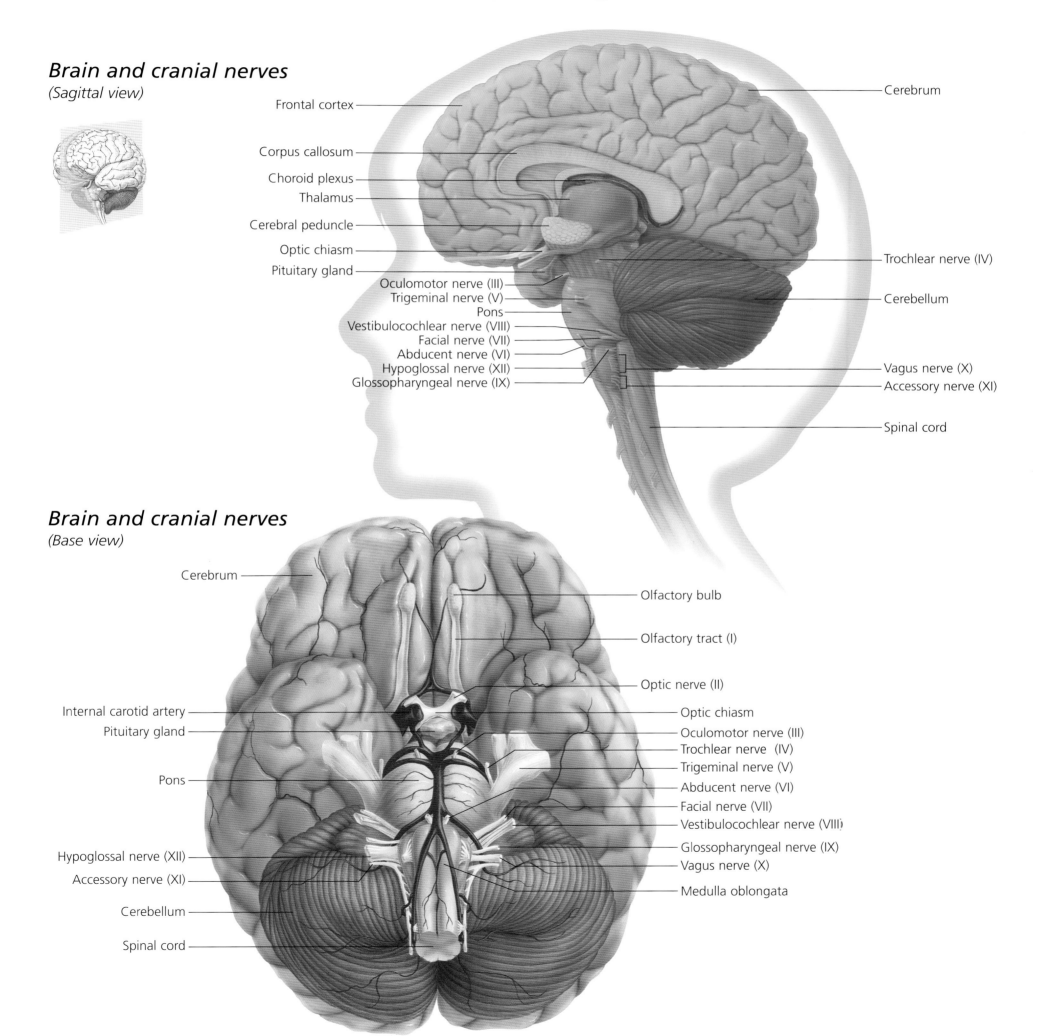

Cerebrum

Frontal cortex

Corpus callosum

Choroid plexus

Thalamus

Cerebral peduncle

Optic chiasm

Pituitary gland

Oculomotor nerve (III)

Trigeminal nerve (V)

Pons

Vestibulocochlear nerve (VIII)

Facial nerve (VII)

Abducent nerve (VI)

Hypoglossal nerve (XII)

Glossopharyngeal nerve (IX)

Trochlear nerve (IV)

Cerebellum

Vagus nerve (X)

Accessory nerve (XI)

Spinal cord

Brain and cranial nerves
(Base view)

Cerebrum

Internal carotid artery

Pituitary gland

Pons

Hypoglossal nerve (XII)

Accessory nerve (XI)

Cerebellum

Spinal cord

Olfactory bulb

Olfactory tract (I)

Optic nerve (II)

Optic chiasm

Oculomotor nerve (III)

Trochlear nerve (IV)

Trigeminal nerve (V)

Abducent nerve (VI)

Facial nerve (VII)

Vestibulocochlear nerve (VIII)

Glossopharyngeal nerve (IX)

Vagus nerve (X)

Medulla oblongata

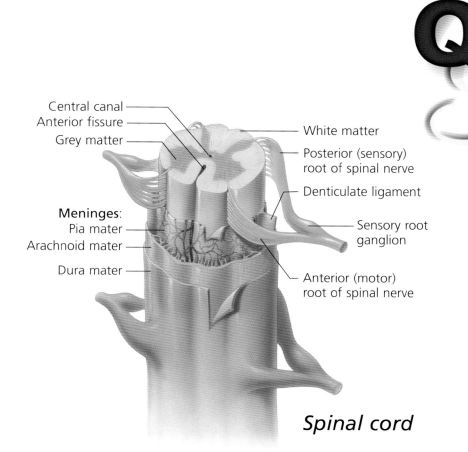

Central canal
Anterior fissure
Grey matter

Meninges:
Pia mater
Arachnoid mater

Dura mater

White matter

Posterior (sensory)
root of spinal nerve

Denticulate ligament

Sensory root
ganglion

Anterior (motor)
root of spinal nerve

Spinal cord

Q & A

What are dermatomes?

A **dermatome** is a specific region of the skin innervated by a pair of cranial or spinal nerves. All the nerve pairs are associated with an area with the exception of cranial nerves C1. The segmented pattern of dermatomes on the body is created by the peripheral nervous system development. The boundaries of a dermatome are not precisely defined, and dermatomes in the appendages can overlap. Because of the correspondence between nerve pairs and specific skin areas, dermatomes may indicate injury to a spinal nerve through a loss of sensation in a specific area.

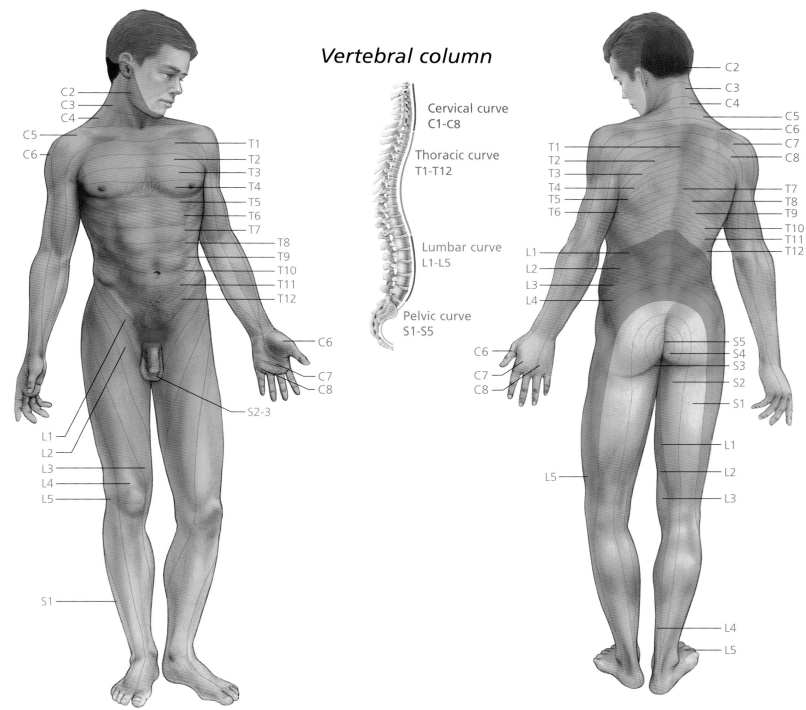

Vertebral column

Cervical curve
C1-C8

Thoracic curve
T1-T12

Lumbar curve
L1-L5

Pelvic curve
S1-S5

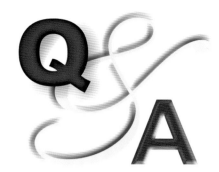

What are the special senses?

The central nervous system (**CNS**) contains thousands of input and output connections between neurons that form dense networks within the brain. Synaptic connections are the tiny spaces between individual neurons where messenger chemicals called **neurotransmitters** are exchanged, initiating new electrical currents within target cells.

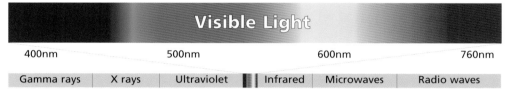

Spectrum

The eye (sight)

The eye is one of the most important of our sensory organs. Often referred to as "the windows to the soul", the eyes are the organs which allow us **stereoscopic vision** (depth perception), an adaptation to the environment which ensured our survival. Our eyes receive a stimulus from light reflected off an object, and photoreceptors in the eye convert this light energy into nerve impulses. Only the visible light portion of the electromagnetic spectrum can trigger these photoreceptors—wavelengths between 400 and 760 nanometers. The brain interprets these signals and gives an accurate analysis of form, light intensity, color and movement.

Rods & cones

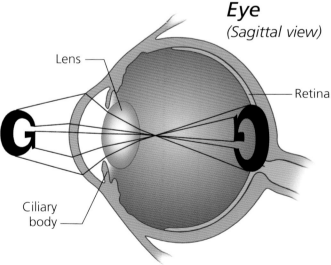

Nerve fibers | Bipolar cells | Rods & cones
Ganglion cells | Pigment layer

Brain
(Inferior view)

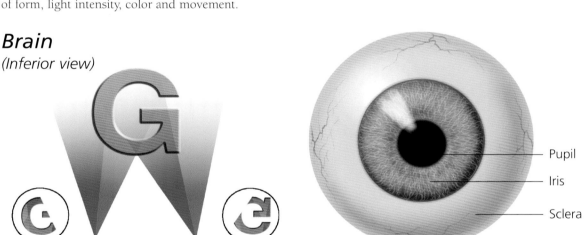

Eye
Retina

Optic nerve
Optic chiasma
Optic tract

Right cerebral hemisphere | Processed information received in the occipital lobe | Left cerebral hemisphere

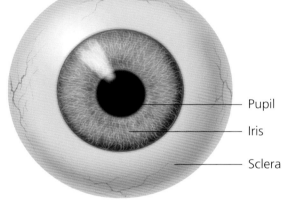

Pupil
Iris
Sclera

Eye
(Sagittal view)

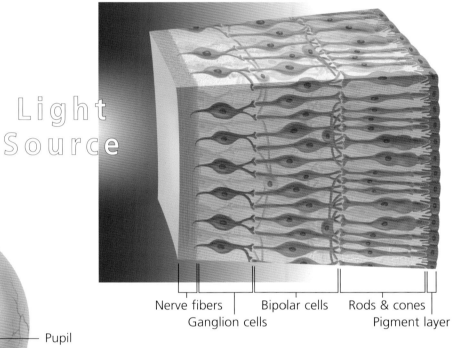

Lens
Retina
Ciliary body

What is a visual field?

The **visual field** is the part of the external world that is projected onto the retina. The cornea and lens focus the right part of the visual field onto the left part of the retina of each eye, and the left part of the visual field is focused onto the right part of the retina of each eye. Within each eye the visual field is projected upside down and reversed because of refraction.

Information about the visual field travels from the retinas to the brain. Information from the right side of the visual field travels from the left halves of both retinas to the left side of the brain. The signals from the left eye cross the **optic chiasma** to reach the right side of the brain. Information about the right side of the visual field hits the right halves of both retinas and travels to the left side of the brain — the signals from the right eye also cross at the optic chiasma. Within the brain, signals travel to areas responsible for perception and eye and body movements.

What is accommodation?

The ability of the eye to keep an image focusing on the retina is called **accommodation**. When light enters the eye, light is **refracted** or focused onto the retina. In order to keep objects that are moving in focus, the eye has to adjust this refraction. It does this by changing the shape of the lens by use of the **ciliary body**. This muscular ring either contracts, making the lens less convex, or relaxes, making the lens more rounded or convex.

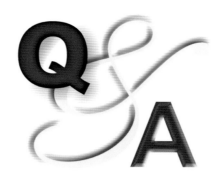

What are the special senses?

The nose (smell)

The sense of smell is called **olfaction**, or the detection of odors. Olfaction depends on specialized chemical receptors, or **chemoreceptors**, located within the olfactory epithelium. These receptors can respond to very small amounts of an **odorant**, a molecule than can be smelled. Humans can detect about 10,000 odors.

Olfactory epithelium

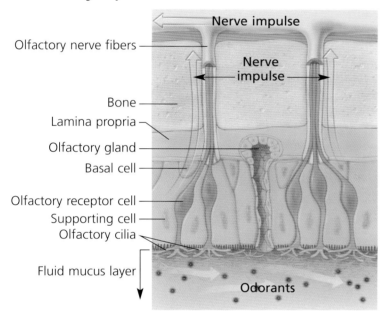

Nerve impulse

Olfactory nerve fibers

Nerve impulse

Bone
Lamina propria
Olfactory gland
Basal cell

Olfactory receptor cell
Supporting cell
Olfactory cilia

Fluid mucus layer

Odorants

Head
(Sagittal view)

Frontal sinus
Olfactory bulb

Olfactory nerve fibers (I)

Sphenoidal sinus

Nasal cavity

Tongue

Oral cavity

The tongue (taste)

Gustation, the sense of taste, gives us information about the food and drink that we consume. **Taste buds** are the primary gustatory receptor, with each taste bud containing chemoreceptors called **gustatory cells**. Four basic tastes have been recognized; sweet, sour, bitter and salty.

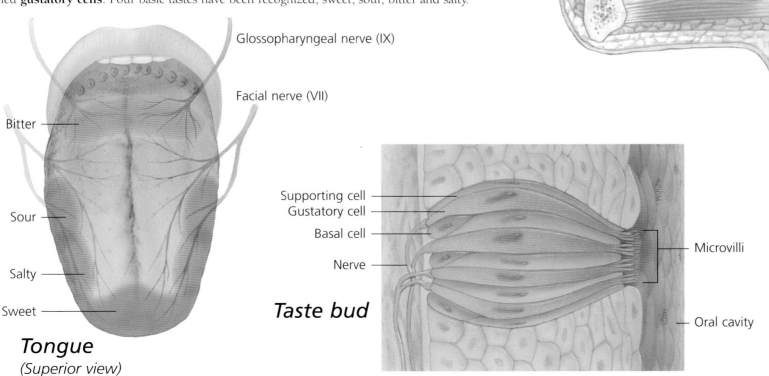

Glossopharyngeal nerve (IX)

Facial nerve (VII)

Bitter

Sour

Salty

Sweet

Tongue
(Superior view)

Supporting cell
Gustatory cell
Basal cell
Nerve

Microvilli

Oral cavity

Taste bud

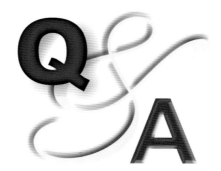

What are the special senses?

The skin (touch)

The skin is a highly elastic organ covering the entire outer surface of the body. It performs numerous functions essential to survival, including prevention of fluid loss from body tissues; protection against environmental toxins and microorganisms; reception of heat, cold and pain sensations; regulation of normal body temperature; and maintenance of calcium levels.

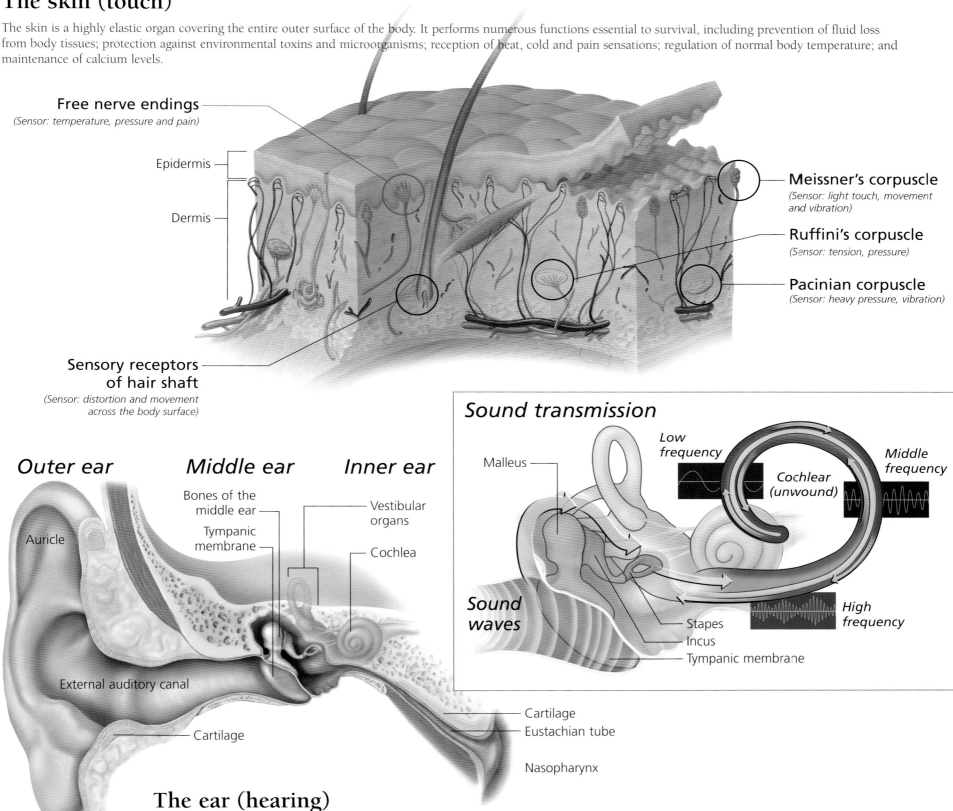

Free nerve endings
(Sensor: temperature, pressure and pain)

Epidermis

Dermis

Sensory receptors of hair shaft
(Sensor: distortion and movement across the body surface)

Meissner's corpuscle
(Sensor: light touch, movement and vibration)

Ruffini's corpuscle
(Sensor: tension, pressure)

Pacinian corpuscle
(Sensor: heavy pressure, vibration)

Sound transmission

Malleus

Low frequency

Middle frequency

Cochlear (unwound)

Sound waves

Stapes
Incus
Tympanic membrane

High frequency

Outer ear

Auricle

External auditory canal

Cartilage

Middle ear

Bones of the middle ear

Tympanic membrane

Inner ear

Vestibular organs

Cochlea

Cartilage
Eustachian tube

Nasopharynx

The ear (hearing)

Air-borne sound waves are collected by the external ear or **auricle** and funneled into the auditory canal, which narrows as it approaches the tympanic membrane, amplifying the waves. The tympanic membrane vibrates in response to the sound waves and transmits vibrations to the bones of the middle ear (**ossicles**). Each of the three linked bones vibrates in a slightly different manner, intensifying the sound as the vibrations are carried across the air-filled cavity to the **oval window**, the entrance to the inner ear. Resulting fluid pressure waves within the inner ear stimulate receptor cells in the organ of Corti, in the central channel of the cochlea. Nerve impulses are carried along the cochlear nerve to the auditory center of the brain and interpreted as sound.

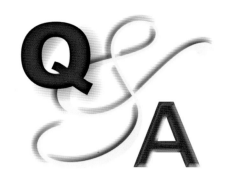

What is epilepsy?

Epilepsy refers to a condition involving recurring or chronic seizures. It is typically defined as two or more seizures occurring at different times without being provoked by fever, exposure to toxic substances or other conditions that could be corrected or avoided. While the origin of most cases of epilepsy is unknown, some cases are known to result from birth injuries (i.e. lack of oxygen); head trauma; inflammation or infection of the brain or membranes; poisoning; and genetic factors.

Functional areas of the brain

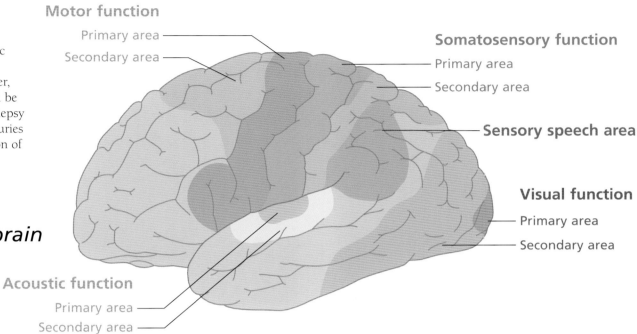

Motor function
Primary area
Secondary area

Somatosensory function
Primary area
Secondary area

Sensory speech area

Visual function
Primary area
Secondary area

Acoustic function
Primary area
Secondary area

What is an epileptic seizure?

The word "seizure" is derived from the Latin word "sacire," which means "to take possession of." An **epileptic seizure** is an episode of uncontrolled, chaotic electrical activity within the brain. There are many types of epilepsy, and the condition can take many forms.

Partial seizures arise from a single area in one cerebral hemisphere of the brain. Resulting symptoms depend on the specific location of the seizure and can range from loss of consciousness to abnormal movement of a single part of the body, such as a hand. Partial seizures can also spread through the cerebral cortex and become more generalized. **Generalized seizures** affect both hemispheres of the brain simultaneously. Symptoms are classified according to different seizure types (see below) ar.d can include a range of symptoms from subtle bilateral motor abnormalities to severe muscle contractions and prolonged unconsciousness.

Tonic-clonic seizure
(Grand mal)

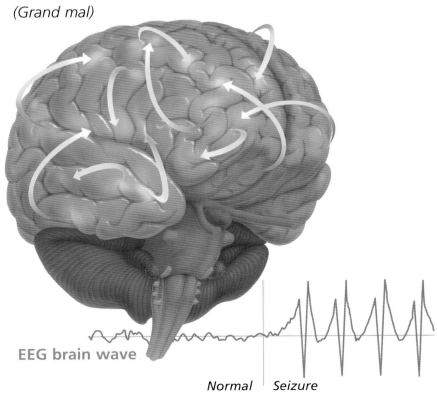

EEG brain wave

Normal | *Seizure*

Complex partial seizure

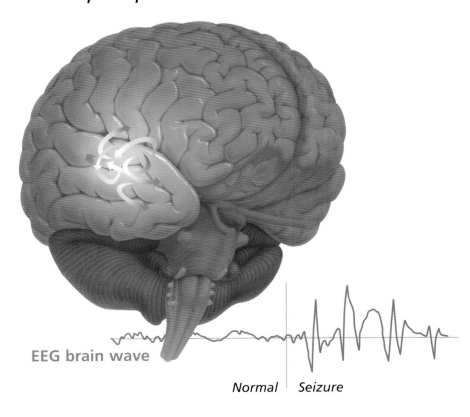

EEG brain wave

Normal | *Seizure*

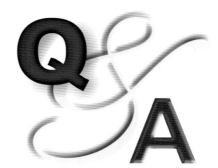

What is stroke?

A **stroke** is a cerebral vascular accident that occurs when blood flow to the brain is suddenly interrupted by a burst blood vessel or a blockage in the brain's blood supply. Nerve cells in the affected part of the brain no longer receive oxygen and nutrients, and the result is temporary or permanent loss of function in the corresponding parts of the body.

Strokes are classified into two major categories:

• **Ischemic** stroke is the most common type, occurring in approximately 80 percent of all cases

• **Hemorrhagic** stroke is present in about 20 percent of stroke cases

Ischemic strokes happen when blood flow to the brain is blocked by clots or fragments that have become lodged within the blood vessels. The origin of the clot determines what type of ischemic stroke has occurred.

Hemorrhagic strokes occur when blood from a ruptured vessel accumulates and compresses surrounding brain tissue, injuring cells and interfering with brain function. The leaking vessel also interrupts oxygen flow to the brain. The amount of bleeding determines the severity of the stroke.

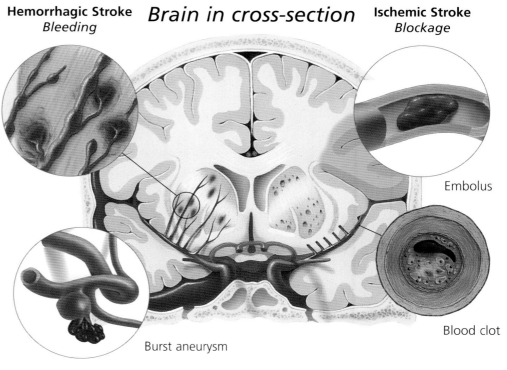

Hemorrhagic Stroke
Bleeding

Brain in cross-section

Ischemic Stroke
Blockage

Area of burst arterioles

Embolus

Burst aneurysm

Blood clot

What are the causes of stroke?

Every type of stroke has a specific physiological cause. In general, however, strokes are frequently caused by underlying medical conditions such as high blood pressure, heart disease, or **atherosclerosis** (narrowing of the arteries). Strokes may also be the result of head injuries, aneurysms or congenital defects in the arteries of the brain.

Meninges of the brain

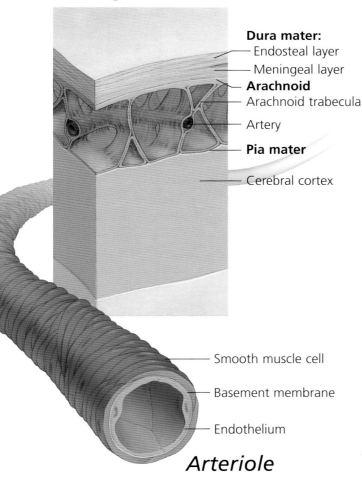

Dura mater:
— Endosteal layer
— Meningeal layer
— **Arachnoid**
— Arachnoid trabecula
— Artery
— **Pia mater**
— Cerebral cortex

— Smooth muscle cell
— Basement membrane
— Endothelium

Arteriole

What are migraines?

The term "migraine" is used to describe a recurring headache syndrome marked by acute sensitivity to environmental and sensory stimuli, such as light, sound, smells and movement. Physiological factors including hormonal fluctuations, excess stress or underlying conditions such as temporomandibular joint disease (TMJ) can also trigger or exacerbate migraines.

Migraine attacks are described as intense, throbbing pain on one or both sides of the head (pain can also begin on one side and switch to the other). The attacks can last anywhere from several hours to several days and recur as infrequently as once or twice a year or as often as several times weekly. Migraine attacks are often incapacitating and may be followed by a period of weakness and fatigue.

What causes migraine headaches?

While the exact cause of migraine headaches is not known, recent evidence suggests that a migraine attack originates as an electrical disturbance in the brain triggered by an outside source, such as food. These changes are believed to affect the release of **serotonin**, an important neurotransmitter that influences many functions in the brain, including pain thresholds and the constriction and dilation of blood vessels. As enlarged blood vessels trigger irritation in surrounding nerve endings, inflammation develops in the protective covering around the brain and spinal cord. The pain of migraine attacks is thought to result from a combination of increased pain sensitivity, vasodilation and inflammation.

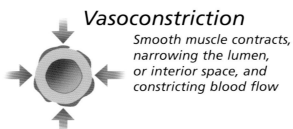

Vasoconstriction
Smooth muscle contracts, narrowing the lumen, or interior space, and constricting blood flow

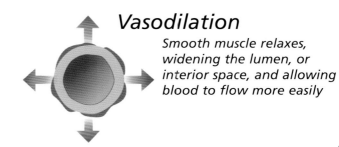

Vasodilation
Smooth muscle relaxes, widening the lumen, or interior space, and allowing blood to flow more easily

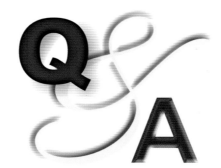

What is depression?

Depression is a significant change in mood that often involves feelings of intense sadness, hopelessness or disinterest in normal daily activities. After anxiety, depression is one of the most common mental health disorders in the United States and can interfere with the ability to work, sleep and eat. Depression may be triggered by traumatic life events or physical health problems and be prolonged or influenced by hereditary and other factors.

Types of depression

There are several types of depression. Depression that persists for more than two weeks is considered **major depression** and includes chronic symptoms such as depressed mood on most days, noticeable loss of pleasure in normal activities, loss of energy, sleeplessness and thoughts of suicide. In **chronic depression** (dysthymia), similar symptoms occur with less intensity but may last for a longer period of time. **Atypical depression** is characterized by excessive eating and sleeping behaviors and may occur simultaneously with other emotional disorders. **Seasonal affective disorder** (SAD) usually occurs during the winter months and is marked by fatigue, overeating and excess sleep patterns.

Serotonin pathways

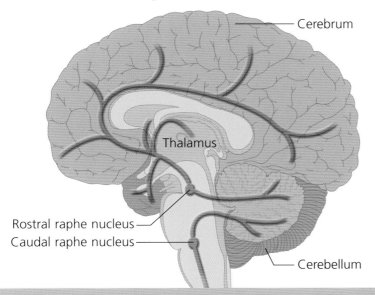

Cerebrum
Thalamus
Rostral raphe nucleus
Caudal raphe nucleus
Cerebellum

Synaptic cleft

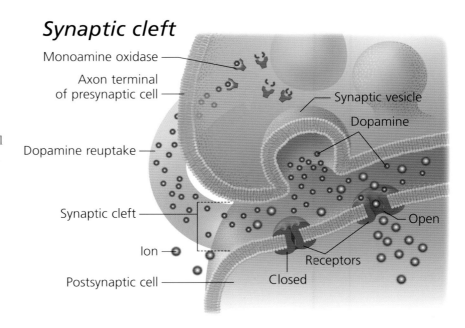

Monoamine oxidase
Axon terminal of presynaptic cell
Synaptic vesicle
Dopamine
Dopamine reuptake
Synaptic cleft
Open
Ion
Postsynaptic cell
Receptors
Closed

What are neurotransmitter pathways?

Neurotransmitters are highly specialized chemical messengers that carry impulses across tiny spaces between **neurons** (nerve cells) in the body. The impulses are sent by the axon of one presynaptic nerve cell and received by the dendrite of the postsynaptic cell. Neurotransmitters are secreted at the contact points between these cells (**synapses**) and trigger receptors on the dendrite to inhibit or excite neural impulses in the target cell. Each type of neurotransmitter (such as **dopamine** and **serotonin**) has unique characteristics that allow it to bind to specific receptor sites on target cells.

Other neurological disorders

Changes in the normal function of the brain, spinal cord or the nerves connected to the CNS may be caused by physical trauma, biochemical imbalances or a variety of other factors. Research and advanced diagnostic techniques are providing new clues into the origin and treatment of many neurological disorders.

Parkinson's disease

- Initiated by degeneration of the area of the brain that produces the neurotransmitter **dopamine**, which regulates motor activity
- Decreasing supplies of dopamine result in progressive weakness, muscle stiffness, tremors and difficulty with posture, motion and speech

Bacterial meningitis

- A dangerous inflammation and infection of the **meninges**, the protective membranes covering the brain and spinal cord
- Caused by bacteria transported through the blood; may also result from an ear or sinus infection or skull fracture
- Symptoms include high fever, chills, headache, stiff neck, nausea, confusion or coma; immediate treatment is required

Alzheimer's disease

- A degenerative condition that gradually destroys nerve cells in the cerebral cortex, impairing movement, cognition and memory
- May be influenced by both genetic and environmental risk factors
- Disease process has been linked to impaired flow of nutrients to neurons; reduced levels of the neurotransmitter acetylcholine; and accumulation of an insoluble protein called **beta amyloid**, which interferes with normal nerve signals and function

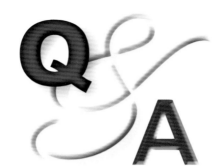

The digestive system

The digestive system, or gastrointestinal tract, is essentially a muscular tube in which intake, digestion and absorption of nutrients takes place. Food, broken down mechanically in the mouth, is propelled through a series of different secretory and absorptive environments. Within these environments, food is digested (broken down) by enzymes into components small enough to be absorbed. The digestive system also stores unabsorbed components until they are ready to be expelled at the end of the gastrointestinal tract.

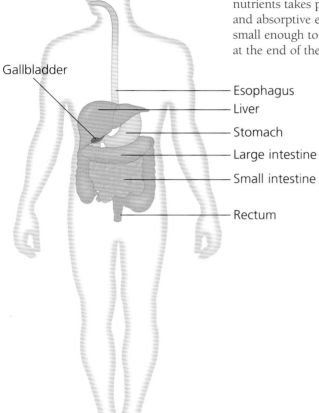

Gallbladder

Esophagus
Liver
Stomach
Large intestine
Small intestine
Rectum

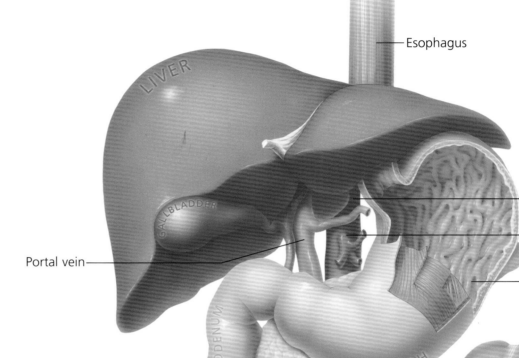

Esophagus

LIVER

GALLBLADDER

Portal vein

Aorta

Celiac trunk

Rugae

DUODENUM

STOMACH

Pancreas

ASCENDING COLON

TRANSVERSE COLON

DESCENDING COLON

JEJUNUM

MESENTERY

ILEUM

SIGMOID COLON

RECTUM

Appendix

External anal sphincter muscles:
Deep
Superficial
Subcutaneous

Levator ani muscle

The mouth & salivary glands

Chewing, the mechanical action of the **teeth** and **tongue**, begins the breakdown of solid food. It greatly increases food's surface area and mixes the food with the secretions of the **salivary glands**, called saliva. Saliva acts like a solvent, cleansing the teeth and dissolving food molecules so they can be tasted. Its enzymes also begin the digestion of starch, a form of carbohydrate, and its mucus lubricates the **pharynx** for swallowing.

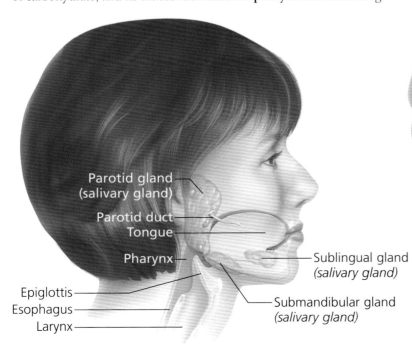

Parotid gland
(salivary gland)
Parotid duct
Tongue
Pharynx
Epiglottis
Esophagus
Larynx

Sublingual gland
(*salivary gland*)

Submandibular gland
(*salivary gland*)

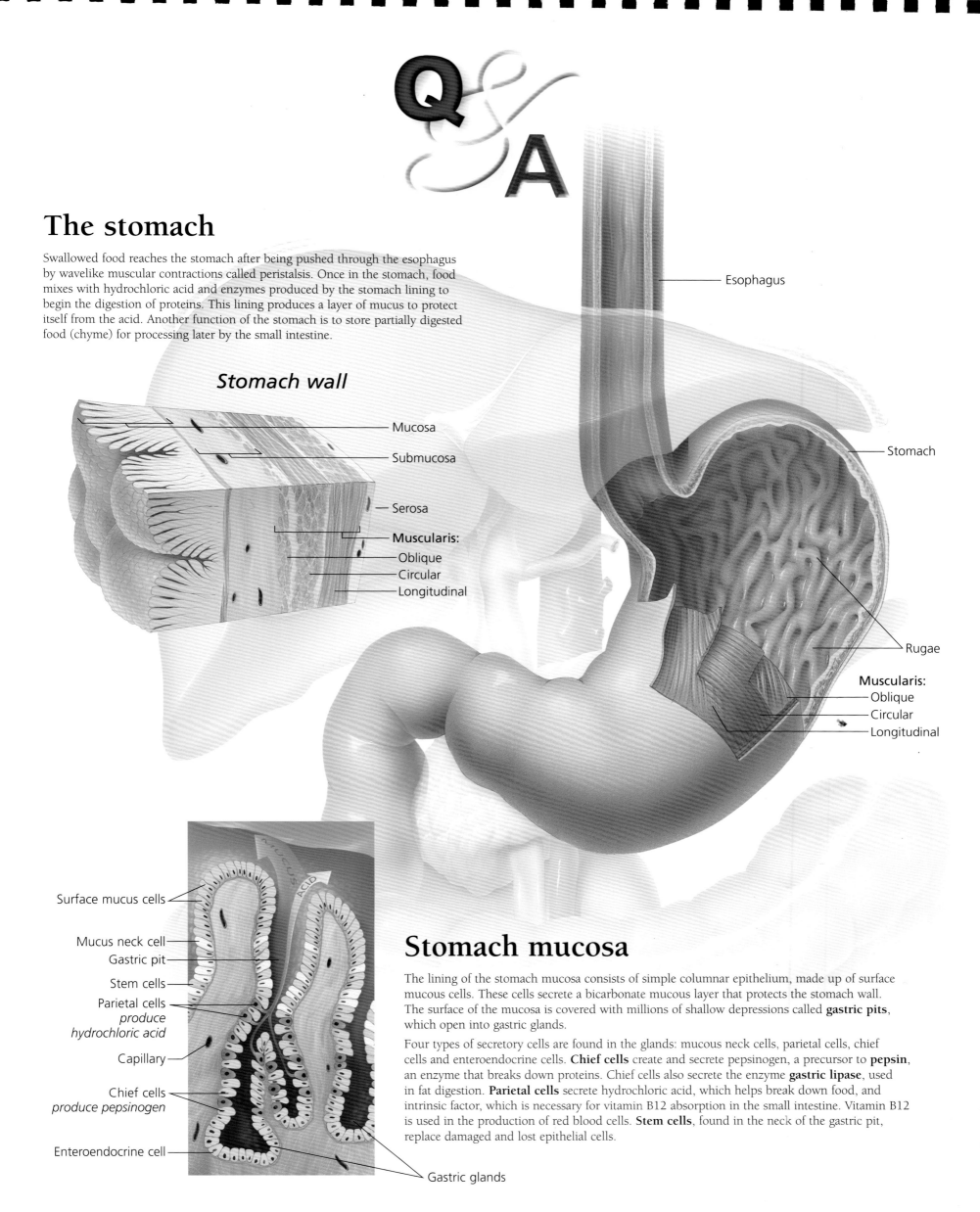

The stomach

Swallowed food reaches the stomach after being pushed through the esophagus by wavelike muscular contractions called peristalsis. Once in the stomach, food mixes with hydrochloric acid and enzymes produced by the stomach lining to begin the digestion of proteins. This lining produces a layer of mucus to protect itself from the acid. Another function of the stomach is to store partially digested food (chyme) for processing later by the small intestine.

Stomach wall

Mucosa
Submucosa
Serosa
Muscularis:
Oblique
Circular
Longitudinal

Esophagus

Stomach

Rugae

Muscularis:
Oblique
Circular
Longitudinal

Surface mucus cells
Mucus neck cell
Gastric pit
Stem cells
Parietal cells *produce hydrochloric acid*
Capillary
Chief cells *produce pepsinogen*
Enteroendocrine cell
Gastric glands

MUCUS
ACID

Stomach mucosa

The lining of the stomach mucosa consists of simple columnar epithelium, made up of surface mucous cells. These cells secrete a bicarbonate mucous layer that protects the stomach wall. The surface of the mucosa is covered with millions of shallow depressions called **gastric pits**, which open into gastric glands.

Four types of secretory cells are found in the glands: mucous neck cells, parietal cells, chief cells and enteroendocrine cells. **Chief cells** create and secrete pepsinogen, a precursor to **pepsin**, an enzyme that breaks down proteins. Chief cells also secrete the enzyme **gastric lipase**, used in fat digestion. **Parietal cells** secrete hydrochloric acid, which helps break down food, and intrinsic factor, which is necessary for vitamin B12 absorption in the small intestine. Vitamin B12 is used in the production of red blood cells. **Stem cells**, found in the neck of the gastric pit, replace damaged and lost epithelial cells.

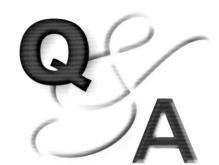

The small intestine

The **small intestine** consists of three areas, the **duodenum**, **jejunum** and **ileum**. Digestion occurs throughout the entire length of the small intestine, accompanied by the **absorption** of the resulting molecules by the intestinal wall. **Villi**, projections of the lining of the small intestine, greatly increase the surface area of the absorptive membrane called the **epithelium**. Each cell of the epithelium has **microvilli**, which further increase this absorptive surface area.

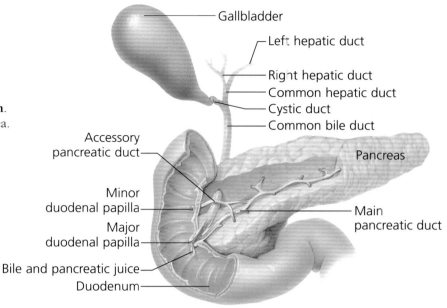

Gallbladder
Left hepatic duct
Right hepatic duct
Common hepatic duct
Cystic duct
Common bile duct
Pancreas
Accessory pancreatic duct
Minor duodenal papilla
Major duodenal papilla
Main pancreatic duct
Bile and pancreatic juice
Duodenum

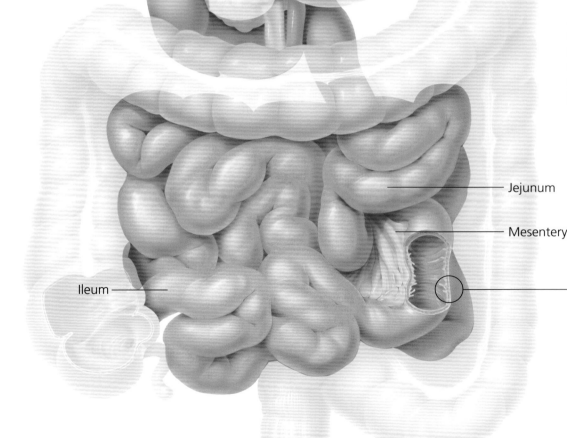

Duodenum

Jejunum

Mesentery

Ileum

Liver, pancreas & gallbladder

After leaving the **stomach**, chyme moves into the **duodenum**, the first part of the **small intestine**, where it is mixed with bile produced by the **liver** and pancreatic juice produced by the **pancreas**. Bile acts as a mixing agent on the chyme while the pancreatic juice containing numerous digestive enzymes further breaks down fats, proteins and carbohydrates. Excess bile is stored in the **gallbladder**.

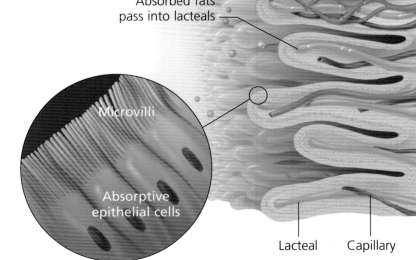

Intestinal lining

Absorbed simple sugars and amino acids pass into capillaries

Epithelium

Villi

Absorbed fats pass into lacteals

Microvilli

Absorptive epithelial cells

Lacteal   Capillary

Absorption

Specialized absorptive cells in the **epithelium** of the small intestine absorb the small molecules produced by digestion. Once absorbed, simple sugars (from carbohydrates) and amino acids (from proteins) enter the **capillaries** of the villi and travel in venous blood from the small intestine to the **liver** via the **portal vein**. This blood is processed by the liver before entering the general circulation. Absorbed fats enter the lymphatic vessels of the villi, called **lacteals**, and circulate in the lymphatic system before eventually entering the blood.

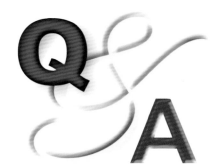

The large intestine

The **large intestine** consists of the **cecum**, the **colon** (**ascending**, **transverse**, **descending** and **sigmoid**) and the **rectum**. As undigested material enters the large intestine, water and electrolytes are absorbed. The remaining waste is stored, formed and expelled.

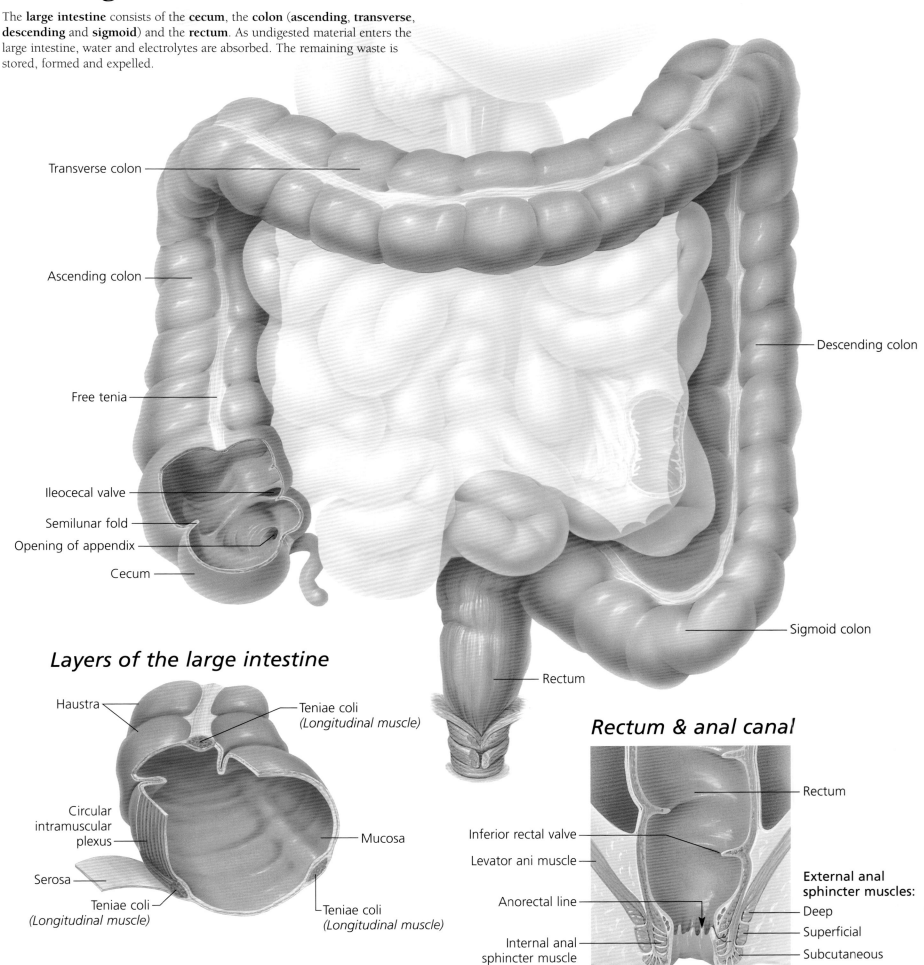

Transverse colon

Ascending colon

Free tenia

Ileocecal valve

Semilunar fold

Opening of appendix

Cecum

Descending colon

Sigmoid colon

Rectum

Layers of the large intestine

Haustra

Teniae coli
(*Longitudinal muscle*)

Circular
intramuscular
plexus

Serosa

Teniae coli
(*Longitudinal muscle*)

Mucosa

Teniae coli
(*Longitudinal muscle*)

Rectum & anal canal

Rectum

Inferior rectal valve

Levator ani muscle

Anorectal line

Internal anal
sphincter muscle

**External anal
sphincter muscles:**

Deep

Superficial

Subcutaneous

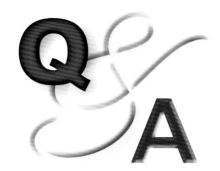

Understanding GERD *(gastroesophageal reflux disease)*

What is GERD?

The most common esophageal disorder is gastroesophageal reflux disease, or GERD, defined as the reflux (regurgitation) of gastric secretions and materials into the esophagus, causing complications and problems. The most common symptom of GERD is heartburn, a burning sensation in the chest that may start in the upper abdomen and radiate into the neck. An estimated 60 million Americans have heartburn at least once a month, with 25% experiencing it daily.

Other symptoms of GERD include the back flow of bitter or sour material into the throat and mouth, especially when lying down or sleeping, and excessive production of saliva (water brash), caused by acid in the esophagus. Less common symptoms are chest pain, difficulty swallowing (dysphagia) and painful swallowing (odynophagia). Inflammation of the esophagus, weight loss and vomiting of blood are symptoms of other problems often associated with GERD. Usually a description of symptoms will allow a physician to establish the diagnosis of GERD.

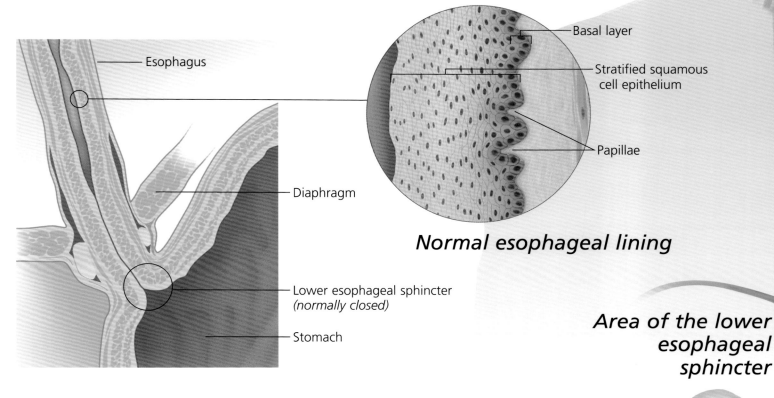

Esophagus

Basal layer

Stratified squamous cell epithelium

Papillae

Diaphragm

Normal esophageal lining

Lower esophageal sphincter *(normally closed)*

Stomach

Area of the lower esophageal sphincter

The esophagus

Under normal circumstances, food passes into the stomach from the esophagus and is prevented from traveling back up the esophagus by the lower esophageal sphincter, which remains tightly closed except when you swallow food. Sometimes the sphincter muscle, at the gastric esophageal junction, becomes weakened and relaxes (opens), allowing acidic stomach contents to move back up the esophagus, producing the symptoms of heartburn.

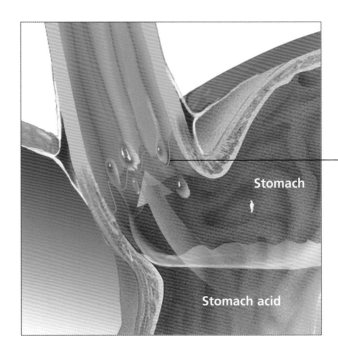

Gastric esophageal junction

Stomach

Stomach acid

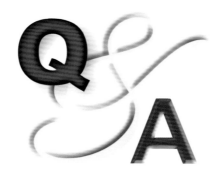

Understanding Barrett's esophagus

The esophageal lining

The **esophagus** is the portion of the digestive canal between the pharynx and stomach. Unlike the lining of the stomach, which has a thin layer of protective mucus, the lining of the esophagus offers a weak defense against stomach acid and other harmful substances. It begins below the tongue and ends at the stomach. At the gastric esophageal junction, the stratified squamous epithelium is abruptly succeeded by simple columnar epithelium with gastric pits and glands.

Esophageal lining with esophagitis

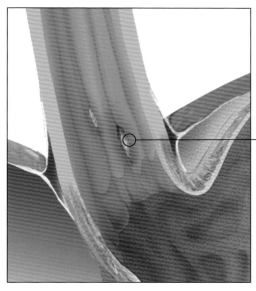

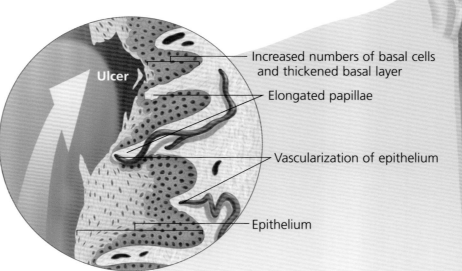

Increased numbers of basal cells and thickened basal layer

Elongated papillae

Ulcer

Vascularization of epithelium

Epithelium

Area of the lower esophageal sphincter

What is esophagitis?

When heartburn becomes more frequent, there is a chance of developing **esophagitis**, an irritation (inflammation) of the esophageal lining caused by stomach acid. If the esophagitis becomes severe, the result can be bleeding and difficulty in swallowing because of a constriction (**stricture**) of the esophagus. Some people with severe esophagitis develop Barrett's esophagus.

Esophageal lining with Barrett's epithelium

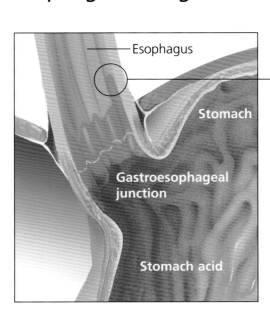

Esophagus

Stomach

Gastroesophageal junction

Stomach acid

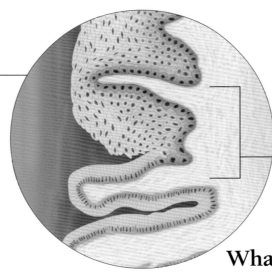

Abrupt change into abnormal specialized columnar epithelium in the esophagus

What is Barrett's esophagus?

In addition to heartburn from a weakened lower esophageal sphincter, many other disorders can result in inflammation of the esophagus. Continual regurgitation of acid from the stomach may damage the normal skin-like lining of the esophagus, which is then replaced by a lining that resembles the lining of the stomach. This new lining usually can resist stomach acid, but inflammation at the upper end of the new lining may cause a stricture, or narrowing, of the interior passageway of the esophagus. Ulcers may occur in the new lining, and can bleed and perforate the esophageal wall. There is a slightly increased risk of cancer occurring in Barrett's esophagus.

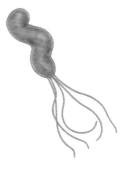

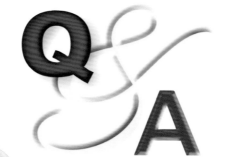

Understanding ulcers

Helicobacter pylori bacteria

Possible causes of ulcers

Ulcers are injuries that occur within the mucosa of the esophagus, stomach, or small intestine as a result of chronic inflammation or exposure to irritants. The most common causes of ulcers in the gastrointestinal system are oversecretion of stomach acid and digestive enzymes, bacterial infection (*Helicobacter pylori*) and the use of non-steroidal anti-inflammatory drugs (NSAIDs). *H. pylori* is most closely linked to the development of duodenal ulcers, while gastric ulcers are more commonly induced by NSAIDs.

Other risk factors for developing ulcers include smoking as well as chronic disorders such as Zollinger-Ellison syndrome, a condition in which high quantities of gastric enzymes are produced by small tumors in the stomach. Psychological stress has been found to increase stomach acid production but has not been clinically proven to cause ulcers. Acute illness, trauma or severe burns can also cause stress ulcers in the gastrointestinal system.

Esophagitis

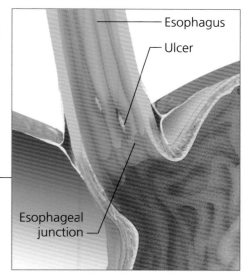

Esophagus

Ulcer

Esophageal junction

Duodenal ulcer

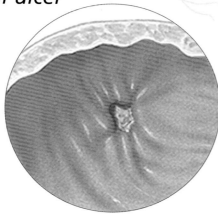

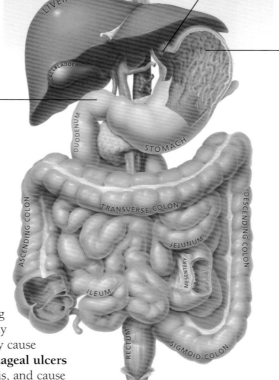

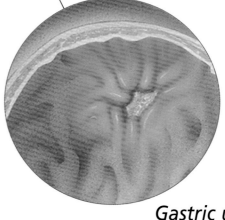

Types of ulcers

The term "ulcer" typically refers to peptic ulcers, which can develop in the **stomach**, the **duodenum** (the upper third of the small intestine just below the stomach), the **jejunum** (below the duodenum) or the **esophagus**. **Duodenal ulcers** are the most common type of ulcer and are associated with symptoms including indigestion, weight gain and stomach pain. **Gastric ulcers** typically occur within the lining of the upper curve of the stomach and may cause gnawing or aching pain as well as gastrointestinal bleeding. **Esophageal ulcers** may lead to a painful inflammatory condition known as esophagitis, and cause difficulty swallowing because of narrowing or stricture within the esophagus.

Gastric ulcers

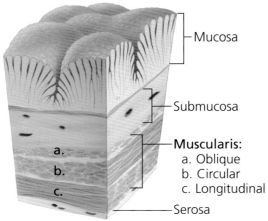

Mucosa

Submucosa

Muscularis:
a. Oblique
b. Circular
c. Longitudinal

Serosa

Normal

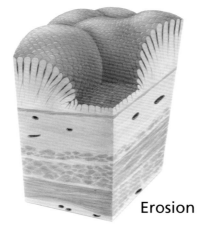

Erosion

Gastric erosions occur when part of the inner layer of the stomach lining is injured by inflammation and exposure to **irritants**, such as NSAIDs, alcohol, caffeine or infection.

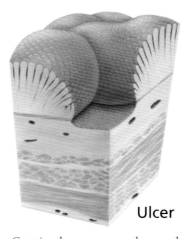

Ulcer

Gastric ulcers are round or oval sores in the lining of the stomach or duodenum caused by chronic exposure to excess stomach acids and **digestive enzymes** (such as hydrochloric acid and pepsin).

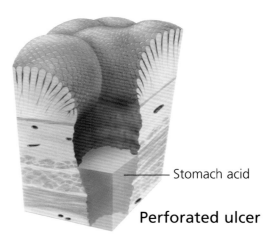

Stomach acid

Perforated ulcer

A small percentage of ulcers lead to perforations in the walls of the stomach or duodenum that open directly into the abdominal cavity.

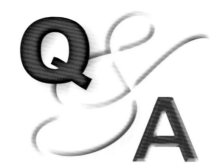

Understanding IBS *(Irritable Bowel Syndrome)*

What is IBS?

Irritable bowel syndrome (IBS) is a functional disorder affecting the large intestine, or colon. With IBS, the colon doesn't work properly, and can lead to chronic and recurrent abdominal discomfort or pain and bowel habit changes. Over the years IBS has been called by different names, such as spastic colon and mucous colitis. Although irritable bowel syndrome has not been shown to lead to other diseases, people with IBS may develop additional disorders.

What causes IBS?

The cause of irritable bowel syndrome is unknown. Since IBS is a functional disorder, there is no infection, inflammation or structural change to be seen. IBS involves a combination of psychological and physiological factors.

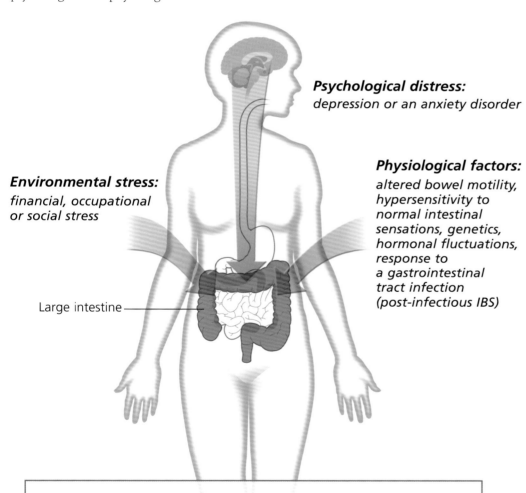

Psychological distress:
depression or an anxiety disorder

Environmental stress:
financial, occupational or social stress

Physiological factors:
altered bowel motility, hypersensitivity to normal intestinal sensations, genetics, hormonal fluctuations, response to a gastrointestinal tract infection (post-infectious IBS)

Large intestine

Symptoms

Normal bowel function varies from one person to the next, and most people have a bowel disturbance from time to time. People with IBS may experience chronic and recurrent abdominal discomfort or pain and bowel disturbances, such as diarrhea (IBS-D), constipation (IBS-C) or alternating diarrhea and constipation (IBS-M).

Colonic movement

Movement through the large intestine is accomplished through the contractions of the longitudinal and circular musculature. Types of movement include peristaltic action, segmentation and mass movement. Movement of feces through the large intestine is slower than through the small intestine, allowing for reabsorption of water.

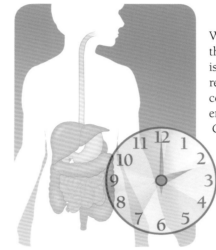

With IBS the rate of movement of the intestinal contents (motility) is abnormal. Rapid motility can result in diarrhea, since the contents are not in the colon long enough for water to be absorbed. Conversely, constipation can result if intestinal contents stay in the colon for a long period of time, allowing too much water to be absorbed.

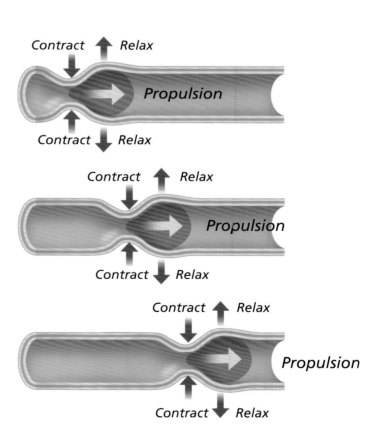

Contract | Relax
Propulsion
Contract | Relax

Contract | Relax
Propulsion
Contract | Relax

Contract | Relax
Propulsion
Contract | Relax

Peristaltic action

Waste material is moved through the colon by a series of coordinated waves of muscle contraction, called peristalsis. The contraction of the muscle behind the waste material pushes it into the next section of colon, where the muscle is relaxed. This section of colon then contracts, pushing the waste into the next (relaxed) colon section, and so on.

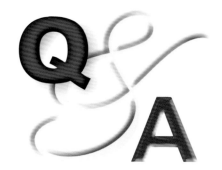

Understanding IBD *(Inflammatory Bowel Disease)*

What is inflammatory bowel disease (IBD)?

The term Inflammatory Bowel Disease (IBD) describes a chronic, relapsing condition characterized by gastrointestinal tract inflammation. Generally, IBD refers to two diseases, **ulcerative colitis** and **Crohn's disease**. While the causes of ulcerative colitis and Crohn's disease remain unknown, heredity and the immune system are believed to be factors. IBD can have complications involving organs outside of the intestines (**extraintestinal**). Some IBD complications are shared by both diseases, while other complications are limited to one or the other. When the determination can't be made (in about ten percent of cases), the condition is called **IBD unspecified** (indeterminate colitis)

What is Crohn's disease?

Crohn's disease is a chronic, relapsing condition characterized by gastrointestinal tract inflammation. The inflammation is not continuous, with areas of normal mucosa separated by inflamed segments. The inflammation can occur anywhere in the gastrointestinal tract, occasionally involving the entire intestinal wall. Complications include small bowel obstruction, fistulas and fissures.

Areas of inflammation

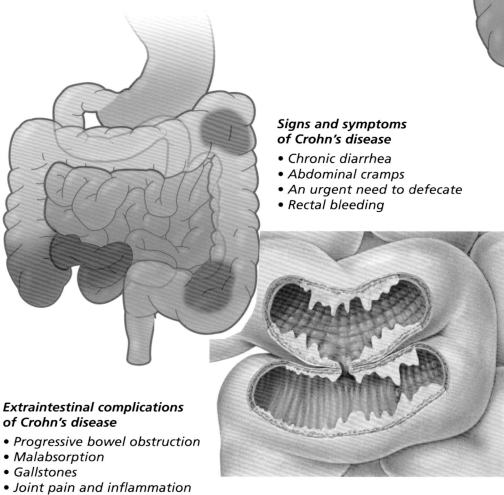

**Signs and symptoms
of Crohn's disease**

- *Chronic diarrhea*
- *Abdominal cramps*
- *An urgent need to defecate*
- *Rectal bleeding*

**Extraintestinal complications
of Crohn's disease**

- *Progressive bowel obstruction*
- *Malabsorption*
- *Gallstones*
- *Joint pain and inflammation*
- *Sacroiliitis (arthritis in the lower back)*
- *Eye inflammation*
- *Skin lesions*

Depending on the length of time and severity of the disease there is an increased risk for colon cancer.

What is ulcerative colitis?

Ulcerative colitis is a chronic condition characterized by gastrointestinal tract inflammation with intermittent worsenings of symptoms separated by remission periods. The inflammation starts in the rectum, and may spread through the large intestine (colon). The inflammation is continuous, involving the mucosal layer of the intestinal wall. If the inflammation only affects the rectum, the condition is termed ulcerative proctitis.

Areas of inflammation

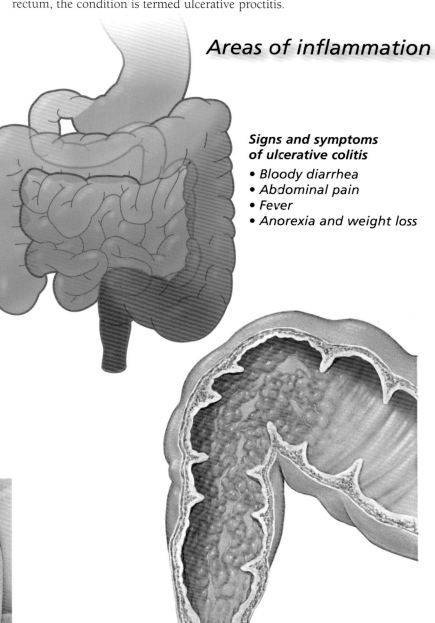

**Signs and symptoms
of ulcerative colitis**

- *Bloody diarrhea*
- *Abdominal pain*
- *Fever*
- *Anorexia and weight loss*

Extraintestinal complications of ulcerative colitis

- *Joint pain and inflammation (arthritis)*
- *Eye inflammation*
- *Skin lesions*

A serious complication, called toxic megacolon, involves the gross dilation of the large intestine, and may require immediate surgery. Depending on the length of time and severity of the disease there is an increased risk for colon cancer.

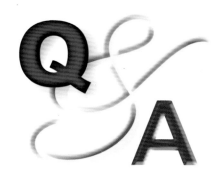

Understanding diarrhea

What is diarrhea?

Diarrhea occurs when the stool becomes loose and watery, usually with an increase in volume and frequency of bowel movements. Normal stool is made up of 60 to 90 percent water. In diarrhea, the stool contains 90 percent water or more. In most cases, this occurs due to a rapid increase in transit time through the large intestine, a process that causes the stool to become excessively watery. Diarrhea can be triggered by a variety of medical conditions, including overactive thyroid and irritable bowel syndrome, by emotional factors such as stress or anxiety, or by certain foods and medications. Different types of diarrhea are commonly caused by specific pathogens (bacteria or viruses).

Close-ups of the intestinal lining

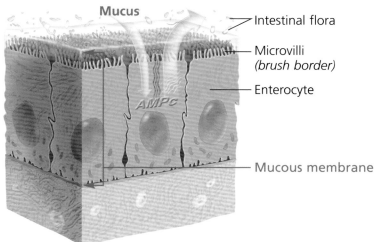

Intestinal lumen — Mucus — Intestinal flora — Microvilli (brush border) — Enterocyte — Mucous membrane — AMPc

Intestinal lining

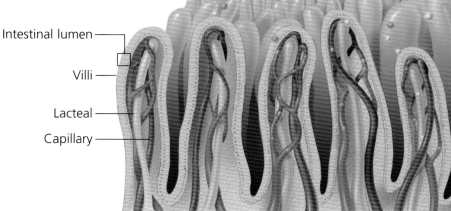

Intestinal lumen — Villi — Lacteal — Capillary

Toxinic (*secretory*) diarrhea

Some bacterial pathogens that cause diarrhea are spread through contaminated food and water. The types of diarrhea caused by these pathogens range from common traveler's diarrhea to cholera. Symptoms usually appear suddenly and can lead to a severe imbalance in bodily fluids that requires prompt treatment. An abundance of watery diarrhea, abdominal cramps and dehydration are common, and nausea and vomiting may also be present.

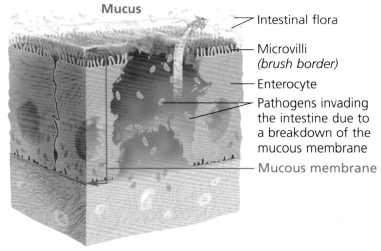

Intestinal lumen — Mucus — Intestinal flora — Microvilli (brush border) — Enterocyte — Pathogens invading the intestine due to a breakdown of the mucous membrane — Mucous membrane

Invasive diarrhea

In some cases of diarrhea, bacterial pathogens such as *E. coli* and *Shigella* attack and invade the protective mucosa (lining) of the intestine, causing cramps, abdominal pain and small, frequent stools containing blood and mucus. Symptoms may be mild or severe and can last from a few days to weeks or more. Pathogens are typically spread by person-to-person contact or through contaminated food.

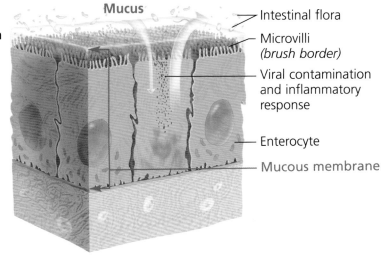

Intestinal lumen — Mucus — Intestinal flora — Microvilli (brush border) — Viral contamination and inflammatory response — Enterocyte — Mucous membrane

Viral diarrhea

Viral pathogens such as Norwalk and rotaviruses cause diarrhea by triggering an inflammatory reaction that reduces the body's ability to absorb water. The sudden imbalance in the volume of water in the intestine results in symptoms including severe cramps, nausea and vomiting. Viruses, one of the leading causes of diarrhea are highly contagious and are usually transmitted through unwashed hands that have been in contact with contaminated feces.

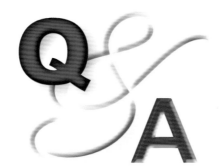

Understanding diseases of the digestive system

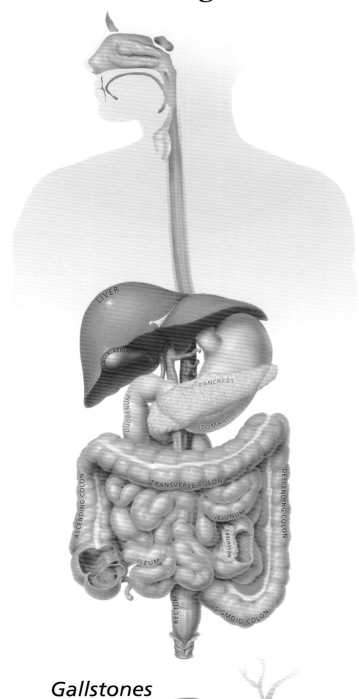

Hiatal hernia

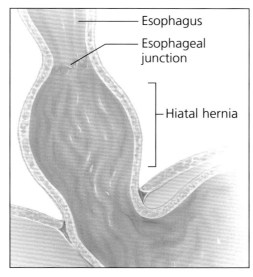

- Esophagus
- Esophageal junction
- Hiatal hernia

Achalasia

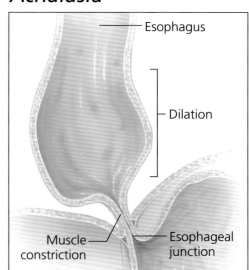

- Esophagus
- Dilation
- Muscle constriction
- Esophageal junction

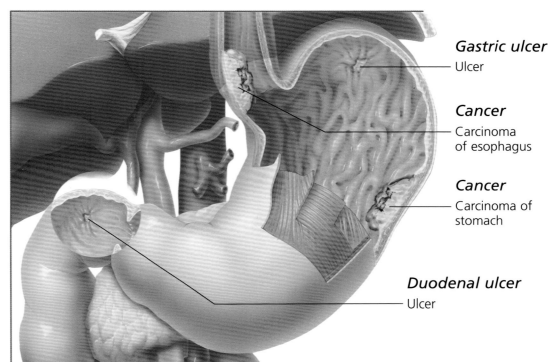

Gastric ulcer
- Ulcer

Cancer
- Carcinoma of esophagus

Cancer
- Carcinoma of stomach

Duodenal ulcer
- Ulcer

Gallstones

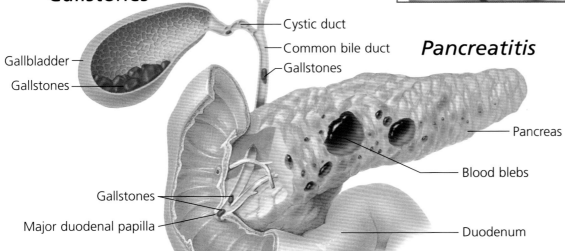

- Cystic duct
- Common bile duct
- Gallstones
- Gallbladder
- Gallstones
- Gallstones
- Major duodenal papilla

Pancreatitis

- Pancreas
- Blood blebs
- Duodenum

Types of gastritis
(inflammation of the stomach wall)

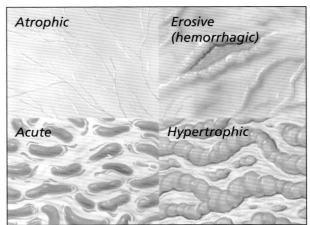

- Atrophic
- Erosive (hemorrhagic)
- Acute
- Hypertrophic

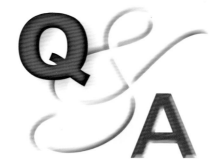

Understanding diseases of the digestive system

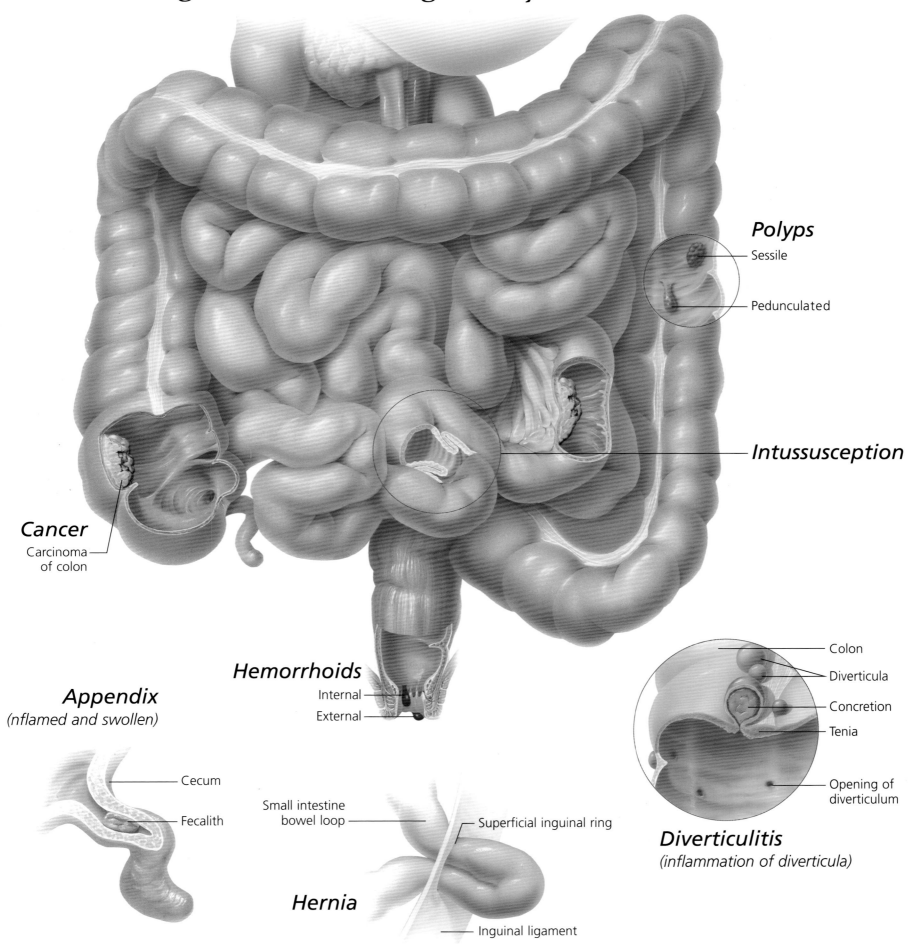

Polyps
- Sessile
- Pedunculated

Intussusception

Cancer
Carcinoma of colon

Hemorrhoids
Internal
External

Appendix
(nflamed and swollen)
- Cecum
- Fecalith

Hernia
Small intestine bowel loop
Superficial inguinal ring
Inguinal ligament

Diverticulitis
(inflammation of diverticula)
- Colon
- Diverticula
- Concretion
- Tenia
- Opening of diverticulum